I0436154

10 Weeks To Better Health

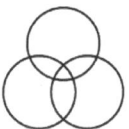

10 Weeks To Better Health

A Plan To Get You Running
And Feeling Great

Eric Prelog

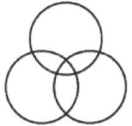

10 Weeks To Better Health: A Plan To Get You Running And Feeling Great.

Copyright © 2012 by Eric Prelog

All rights reserved. Printed in the United States of America. Unless otherwise noted, all material comes from Eric Prelog. No part of this book may be used or reproduced without written permission, except in the case of brief quotations. For information, please email Eric Prelog at eric@totalwellnesshelp.com.

Disclaimer

This book is written for informational purposes only and should not be considered advice. The author believes that most USDA and medical recommendations are not necessarily based in science, and urges the reader to seek the advice of a doctor who is familiar with *all* the nutritional literature before beginning any diet or exercise program.

Welcome

Do you want to become healthier and experience an improved sense of well-being? Would you like to stop worrying about your blood pressure and weight? Have you thought about running but decided against it because of running's bad reputation for injury?

The Plan in this short book is a holistic 10 week schedule designed to improve your overall health and, in the process, take you from someone who can walk 3 miles to someone who can jog or run three miles. The point is not to be able to run three miles, but the improvement of your physical, mental, and spiritual well-being. This is not a program to enhance your running performance. The journey you are beginning will involve changing your perspective about eating, sleeping, exercising, and running. You will become healthier, not only in your body but in your mind and spirit as well.

Many people treat themselves with ice cream, a day off training, a night of drinking, or other more tangible reward after a workout. The perspective of this Plan encourages you to view improved health and the training itself as the reward.

Gratitude

Some people call it god; some call it spirit. I call these cycles within cycles the Universe or the Design. I owe all that I am to the Universe, which equipped me to think, to understand, to know, and to move. It is the Universe from which we come. It is the Universe to which we go. It is in the Universe that we have our being. All blessings in life come from the Universe.

Asher, you and your running have been an inspiration for me on the trail. When I'm discouraged, I think about the unofficial half-marathon you ran barefoot, and I smile. Abby, Katie, Gracie, Maddie – You have all inspired me to be better than I am, to grow, to learn. Mom, Dad, as always. Tallie, spirit in you silences the "why?" and amplifies the "why not?"

There are my brothers, of course - Joel, Andy, and Sam, close friends all. Last, I'm grateful for those who have listened and tried some of my ideas for improving health. Thank you for your willingness to try new things.

PART I

Behind The Plan

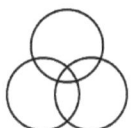

Mindfulness

In the modern world, we awaken to an alarm clock, hurry into the shower, grab a cup of coffee, and jostle our way to work, where we stress as if we're fighting for survival. After work, we rush home, take the kids to the activity-of-the-day, get some dinner from a box in the pantry or a boxy store in the shopping center, watch a few minutes of bad news, have a glass of wine[*] to de-stress, and go to bed.

This way of life isn't necessarily good for us. We have developed very sophisticated mechanisms to deal with the stress of being chased by a sabre-toothed cat or the danger of being gored by a walrus. These were rare events in our history, but the pace of society encourages us to feel like we're in danger at all times.

During times of stress, our perception narrows to a sharp focus, and our breathing becomes shallow. Our bodies release cortisol (and adrenaline if it's really bad), and our spirits become stifled by the imminent danger we're facing. This fast-paced life over-stimulates our sympathetic nervous system, inducing the fight-or-flight survival responses that have helped us move to the top of the food chain.

The stress response is fun sometimes! Riding rollercoasters or bungee jumping can really break up the tedium of a long summer! These occasional activities are not the problem. The problem is that we're not adapted to be in a constant state of fighting for our lives. On the contrary, we're adapted to slowing down and taking it easy most of the time. In fact, our bodies, minds, and spirits were meant for a life consisting primarily of relaxation, with some stress

---

[*] Alcohol dehydrates your body. Wine contains some great anti-oxidants, but alcohol is an oxidative agent. In general, more than one glass is probably not a good idea.

thrown in now and then for good measure. When we're relaxed, we grow, learn, and appreciate life. Ferris Bueller said it best, "Life moves pretty fast. If you don't stop and look around once in a while, you could miss it."

This stopping and looking around is called *mindfulness*. You don't need to be a yoga guru or a zen monk to practice mindfulness. All you need to do is take a few minutes each day to be still and look around. It can be as easy as sitting on the edge of your bed for a few minutes when you first wake up or taking a walk around the block when you get home from work. Simply be where you are, without worrying about problems or what you've got to do. Pay attention to your thoughts as they enter your mind, and let them go. Be aware of your emotions and stresses relative to your world. How do things look? How do you feel? Practice this, and you will experience an expanded awareness of self and surroundings.

Mindfulness will help to create a more optimistic outlook, abundant with opportunity instead of fraught with danger. It will encourage a spirit of appreciation for all that is in your life. Sunsets will become more beautiful. Work will become less stressful. Connection with your world will become more important. Your spirit will grow.*

---

*Please see the Appendix for a discussion of the interdependence of Spirit, Body, and Mind.

Effects of exercise

Many of the positive effects of exercise are well documented. Only a few of them are listed here. When exercising regularly with moderate intensity, you can expect to experience changes in some or all of these areas:

-Mood level and stability throughout the day
-Immune system will be stronger[*]
-Energy level will increase
-Reduction in blood pressure
-Reduction in Type II diabetes risk
-Reduction in heart disease risk
-Sleep quality
-Enhanced mental clarity
-Increased libido

Some of these are benefits that you may not be able to get from a change in diet or lifestyle. Nobody knows all the benefits of regular exercise. I'll just say, look at us: With our joints, muscles, and amazing coordination, we are built to move with a greater variety of motion than any other organism yet discovered. Exercising is good for us. It's one of the things we are built to do.

Running history

This booklet focuses on running as the primary exercise, so some history is in order. Anthropologist Marvin Harris opens his book *Our Kind* with the statement, "In the beginning was the foot." He justifies this pedestrian statement by describing how our ancestors would "persistence hunt" everything and anything. Persistence

---

[*]Over training, or constantly training at high intensity will weaken the immune system. Some symptoms of over training are constant exhaustion or soreness, persistent colds, increased allergy problems, rashes, depression.

hunting is the process of chasing down prey on foot. He goes on to explain some of the physiological adaptations that enable humans to outrun *any* land animal over distance. (It's no wonder all the other animals are afraid of humans!)

Chasing down prey on foot is one thing. No more than 6 miles is required for most animals. But we can go much further than that. With sufficient training, the sophisticated shock absorption system of our legs and feet allows us to run for days, literally, without significant injury or wear-and-tear on our bodies.

How can this be, you say, since running is hard on the ankles, knees, and hips? It comes down to form, and while a discussion of proper running form is outside the scope[*] of this book, the easy way to run with proper form is to run barefoot. Simply kick off your shoes and run down the sidewalk or street, landing on the balls of your feet in such a way that you don't jar your knees or break your heels. You'll not be far from perfect running form.

Running is not the only exercise that's good or natural for us. We are also able to lift heavy things, climb, stretch, reach, throw, catch, and on and on. All of these activities are beneficial to our physical, mental, and spiritual well-being.

While humans have been out-running everything on feet, we have also been out-eating them in terms of variety. We can and do survive on practically any non-poisonous thing that grows in nature, from the blubber of arctic seals to the inner bark of certain rain-forest trees, to dandelions, crawdads, and insects. While roasted grasshoppers and gopher stew have a certain appeal, I'll go

---

[*]For a full treatment of proper running form, see Danny Dreyer's book, *Chi Running*, Touchstone, 2009.

out on a limb and say that most readers probably prefer the foods we find in our neighborhood grocery store.

Food

Speaking of the grocery store, some of the most important changes you'll be making in this Plan will be to your diet. For many years, the USDA wanted you to believe that the food pyramid was the healthy way to eat, that grains and grain products form the foundation of good health. The fact is that the food pyramid shows which crops are most heavily supported by lucrative USDA subsidies. It is no more than a money trail, and a diet based on governmental subsidies simply does not promote well-being. Their new "Food Plate" of recent years is not an improvement, and it doesn't go far enough in promoting a diet rich in natural fats and colorful vegetables. They still insist that getting 25 percent of our sustenance from grains is a good idea. Grains, which come from grasses, are great food for ruminants, bugs, and birds, but humans lack the enzymes[*] needed to sufficiently digest some of the phytates, lectins, and proteins (like gluten) found in them.

The best food for us is that which grows naturally: vegetables, animals, fish, fruit, insects, nuts,[†] etc. It is debated whether we should be eating cooked food or raw, but the one truth that is NOT at issue is that we should not be eating packaged or refined foods. Who ever saw a Twinkie or a Banquet TV dinner growing from a tree?

A diet high in refined foods and processed carbohydrates contributes[‡] to metabolic syndrome, heart disease, stroke, cancer,

---

[*]Ruminants (cud-chewers) are able to deal with the anti-nutrients found in grains.
[†]Many nuts have a great nutrient profile, but they still contain some anti-nutrients.
[‡]Some experts even say that it *causes* these dis-eases.

diabetes, and most of the other modern plagues on human health. So the insect and rodent comments probably didn't convince you to give up that hot fudge sundae, but maybe Type II diabetes will.

On this plan, you will be eating vegetables, a variety of meats, and a little fruit and nuts. We'll be taking our cues from the natural world. Fruit has a short growing season and does not preserve well, so that will be the smallest part of our diet. Feel free to eat whatever can be grown outside, locally. In a greater amount than fruit, you will consume nuts and vegetables, especially squash (a nutritional powerhouse), cruciferous plants like broccoli and cauliflower, and whatever happens to be in season. In a equal or greater amount than vegetables, you'll be eating fish, meat, and poultry, as these were preservable and available to our ancestors year-round. Try to consume organic foods because they put fewer chemicals into your body and the environment and are more likely to be sustainably farmed.

You won't be too concerned how much food you eat. Mindfully, you'll eat slowly, until you're satisfied but not stuffed. Your blood sugar should stabilize at a lower level (hopefully under 90), and since you're not eating much sugar, your body won't store extra calories as fat.[*] Quality food is important and is defined as that food which grows on its own in nature and doesn't come in a package. A good rule of thumb is that if it would still be edible after two weeks on your counter, it's not edible at all.

Water, water, water!!!

The importance of water cannot be over-emphasized. After oxygen, water is the most critical nutrient in our diet. Drink lots of

---

[*]For a discussion of metabolism and the role sugar plays in fat storage, see Gary Taubes, *Why We Get Fat And What To Do About It.*

it, whether or not you're exercising. Without sufficient water, you won't feel as well; you won't lose weight as well; you won't think as well. It is the basis for all bodily functions.

PART II

The Plan

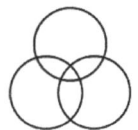

Part II focuses on the specifics of the plan to get you from your couch to running your first 5k. It is a ten week plan to help you clean up your insides and put you on the road to improved fitness through running.

Preparation for the workout – Week 1

Week 1 – This is your Preparation Week. You'll want to spend a week recording how you feel when you wake up and when you go to bed. Writing in a journal will help you understand your progress. It will help you gauge your peace level, which you should find increases with this plan.

In addition to writing in your journal, you'll also want to pick up a few minor supplies. Here's what you'll need:

1. A desire to become more healthy
2. Workout clothes
3. The ability to walk 3 miles without stopping[*]
4. A stopwatch or countdown timer
5. Water bottle

Practice shopping in the produce section of your neighborhood grocery or health food store. Practice slowing down…when you drive, when you do chores, when you work, if possible. Start building empty space into your day for contemplation or just for peace and quiet. Turn off the television. Get away from your email and phone. Watch the sunset or the sunrise. Stand outside in the rain. Practice reading the ingredients on everything you buy. Most

---

[*]If you cannot walk three miles without stopping, begin walking every day. Gradually increase your distance until you reach three miles. Then begin this plan.

13

of the food you'll be eating won't even have a label. Pick up a fat/carb/fiber counting book.[*] Learn to drink lots of water.

Day 7, Pre-Day – The last day of Week 1 is Pre-Day. On Pre-Day, drink lots of water and get at least 7 hours of sleep. Eat well-rounded meals consisting of protein, fat[†], and perhaps some berries or an apple, for example. Drink water.

<u>Beginning the workout – Week 2</u>
Day 8 – Drink a large glass of water first thing in the morning. Start your day with some peace and quiet, taking time to put the upcoming stresses in their proper place. Eat your breakfast, which should be similar to the one you ate on your Pre-Day. Wait at least 1 hour after eating. On Day 8, just walk three miles, without stopping, so that you become familiar with that distance. Drink water during your walk. Note your starting and stopping times.[‡]

After your walk, drink water, and rest for a few minutes in peace and quiet. Write in your journal. Practice mindfulness. Do things look different than they did before? Is your mind quieter? Do you feel exhausted or more alive?

Eat a well-rounded lunch consisting of protein, fat, and some lower-sugar vegetables. Drink water. Eat a well-rounded dinner consisting of fat, protein, and vegetables. Drink water.[§] Get to bed at a decent hour so you can get a full night of sleep.

---

[*]A good website for nutrition data is http://www.nutritiondata.self.com.
[†]Any kind of unprocessed animal or vegetable fat will do. No hydrogenated or other processed fat should be consumed.
[‡]You will gauge your progress in part by how long it takes to cover 3 miles.
[§]Do you get the idea that drinking water is important?

Day 9 – On Day 9, you'll have a low-impact, non-running workout. You'll want to begin developing the habit of switching between low and high impact workouts. Yoga, pilates, swimming, bicycling are all great low-impact activities. Start your workout with a half-mile walk. Drink lots of water. Journal. Eat well-balanced meals. Get at least seven hours of sleep.

Day 10 – On Day 10, you'll walk the first half-mile. The next two miles will go like this: You'll walk five minutes, then jog one minute. * Repeat, alternating between walking and jogging until you have about a half to a quarter mile remaining. Then walk the remainder of your course. Note your starting and stopping times. Drink water during your workout.

When you've completed your workout, rest for about ten minutes. Some people like to stretch after a workout. If you do, rest after stretching. Within thirty minutes after resting, consume some fat, protein, and fruit. Avocado, nuts, and some pineapple would be perfect. Or some eggs, cheese (if you're not lactose-intolerant), and an apple. The sugars in the fruit will help your body use the fat, and they will also work with the protein to replenish and repair the muscles you have just stressed, speeding your recovery.

For the rest of the day, eat well-balanced meals as on the Pre-Day, drinking plenty of water. Make sure your remaining meals contain plenty of fat and protein. Pay attention. Journal. Continue to practice mindfulness. Get lots of sleep that night.

---

*Jog slowly, maintaining the ability to hold a conversation. If you're training alone, practice breathing like this: breathe out for three steps, breathe in for two. If you cannot maintain your conversation or breathing rhythm, you're pushing too hard. Your speed, ease, and level of fitness will improve as you relax into this training.

Day 11 – Day 11 will be a low-impact workout as on Day 9. Drink water before, during, and after your workout. Eat well. Journal about how you're feeling. Practice mindfulness. Sleep at least seven hours.

Day 12 – Day 12 will mirror Day 10. Walk the first half-mile. Then walk/jog according to the same 5/1 ratio you used on Day 10, maintaining breathing or conversation. Repeat until a half to a quarter mile remains. Then walk the remainder of your course. Drink water during your workout.

After the workout, drink water. Rest. Pay attention. Practice mindfulness.

Within 30 minutes after resting, eat as on Day 10. You'll want to develop a gratitude habit of replenishing your body after it has depleted itself for you.

The remainder of Day 12 will follow the pattern of Day 10. Eat well-rounded meals. Drink water. Journal. Practice mindfulness. Sleep at least seven hours.

Day 13 – This day will be almost identical to Day 11. It will be another low-impact workout. Drink water before, during, and after your workout. Eat well. Journal. Practice mindfulness. Sleep seven hours.

Day 14 – Rest. Eat. Take a few minutes of quiet time. Journal. Practice mindfulness. Sleep.

At this point, you will have completed the first two weeks of The Plan. Here's what you've done so far.

Week 1

The first week was mostly focused on how you felt when you woke up and when you went to bed. This was the beginning of mindfulness. The Pre-Day was also focused on nutrition and mindfulness. The first week has begun to develop the new habits of mindfulness and self-care.

Week 2

The second week added the activity focus of a daily workout. You maintained your nutrition and mindfulness during this week while beginning to exercise regularly.

Week 3[*]

The third week will continue the pattern begun in Week 2. You will maintain your nutrition, journaling, and mindfulness, while you continue to develop the habit of exercise. You're now getting into the flow of The Plan.

---

[*]The schedule in The Plan can be adjusted if it's too aggressive for your fitness level. Just add a day each of jogging, low-impact, and rest. It would then become a 10-day workout cycle. Alternatively, you could take two weeks for every week of The Plan, or change a low-impact day into a rest day. Your options are limitless. Try to be mindful of how you're feeling, and adjust accordingly.

Day 15 – Three mile course. Begin with a half mile walking. The next two miles will go like this: You'll walk 5 minutes, then jog 2 minutes. Drink water. Rest. Journal. Eat to replenish.

Day 16 – Low-impact workout day. Journal.
Day 17 – Repeat of Day 15.
Day 18 – Repeat of Day 16.
Day 19 – Repeat of Day 15.
Day 20 – Repeat of Day 16.
Day 21 – Rest. Compare your starting and stopping times from Day 10 to those on Day 21, and note your improvement.

By now you have completed the first three weeks of The Plan and are well on your way to developing healthy self-care habits. You may be feeling your connection to the world around you deepening. You may feel your compassion for others growing, too. Ironically, these are natural outgrowths of taking better care of yourself. You may feel a desire to help others, volunteer your time or join a spiritual congregation. Your improved physical and mental wellness are now beginning to improve your spiritual wellness!

<u>Week 4 and beyond</u>

The table in Part III covers the remaining weeks of The Plan. During these weeks, you will walk your half-mile BEFORE beginning the workout. Remember to maintain your mindfulness, nutrition, journaling, and relaxed pace during the remainder of The Plan.

After completing all 10 weeks of The Plan, you should be ready for your 5k run. Compare your starting and stopping times from Day 10 to those at the end of your ten weeks, and note the improvement you've made. You can be proud of that!

Take a couple days off, and then go for it. Do not be afraid to begin by walking a little or to walk during the run. Rest is important, even in the middle of a race.

After your successful 5k run, don't stop! Living according to The Plan will help you maintain a high level of physical, mental, and spiritual wellness throughout your life. Continue to grow. Continue to eat, exercise, and live mindfully. Continue to live healthfully. Continue to LIVE!

PART III

The Plan In A Nutshell

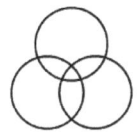

The following table contains The Plan in a layout that should be easy to understand and follow. Continue to journal regularly after the first week.

Week	Day	Activity*	Activity Details
1	1	None	Journal
	2	None	Journal
	3	None	Journal
	4	None	Journal
	5	None	Journal
	6	None	Journal
	7	Pre-day	Pre-day
2†	8	5 / 1	Walk first 1/2 mile of the 3
	9	L I	Yoga/swimming/weights
	10	5 / 1	Walk first 1/2 mile of the 3
	11	L I	Yoga/swimming/weights
	12	5 / 1	Walk first 1/2 mile of the 3
	13	L I	Yoga/swimming/weights
	14	Rest	N/A
3‡	15	5 / 2	3.5 total miles
	16	L I	Yoga/swimming/weights
	17	5 / 2	3.5 total miles
	18	L I	Yoga/swimming/weights
	19	5 / 2	3.5 total miles
	20	L I	Yoga/swimming/weights
	21	Rest	N/A

*The activity column is "Minutes walk / Minutes jog," or "L I" for Low Impact activity.
†Walk ½ mile to warm up. This is the first ½ mile of the 3 mile distance for Week 2.
‡Walk ½ mile to warm up. This is BEFORE the 3 mile distance in Week 3.

23

Week	Day	Activity	Activity details
4	22	4 / 3	3.5 total miles
	23	L I	Yoga/swimming/weights
	24	4 / 3	3.5 total miles
	25	L I	Yoga/swimming/weights
	26	4 / 3	3.5 total miles
	27	L I	Yoga/swimming/weights
	28	Rest	N/A
5	29	3 / 4	3.5 total miles
	30	L I	Yoga/swimming/weights
	31	3 / 4	3.5 total miles
	32	L I	Yoga/swimming/weights
	33	3 / 4	3.5 total miles
	34	L I	Yoga/swimming/weights
	35	Rest	N/A
6	36	2 / 5	3.5 total miles
	37	L I	Yoga/swimming/weights
	38	2 / 5	3.5 total miles
	39	L I	Yoga/swimming/weights
	40	2 / 5	3.5 total miles
	41	L I	Yoga/swimming/weights
	42	Rest	N/A

Week	Day	Activity	Activity details
7	43	1 / 5	3.5 total miles
	44	L I	Yoga/swimming/weights
	45	1 / 5	3.5 total miles
	46	L I	Yoga/swimming/weights
	47	1 / 5	3.5 total miles
	48	L I	Yoga/swimming/weights
	49	Rest	N/A
8	50	2 / 7	3.5 total miles
	51	L I	Yoga/swimming/weights
	52	2 / 7	3.5 total miles
	53	L I	Yoga/swimming/weights
	54	2 / 7	3.5 total miles
	55	L I	Yoga/swimming/weights
	56	Rest	N/A
9	57	1 / 8	3.5 total miles
	58	L I	Yoga/swimming/weights
	59	1 / 6	3.5 total miles
	60	L I	Yoga/swimming/weights
	61	1 / 8	3.5 total miles
	62	L I	Yoga/swimming/weights
	63	Rest	N/A

Week	Day	Activity	Activity details
10	64	1 / 10	3.5 total miles
	65	L I	Yoga/swimming/weights
	66	2 / 15	3.5 total miles
	67	L I	Yoga/swimming/weights
	68	1 / 15	3.5 total miles
	69	L I	Yoga/swimming/weights
	70	Rest	N/A

Appendix

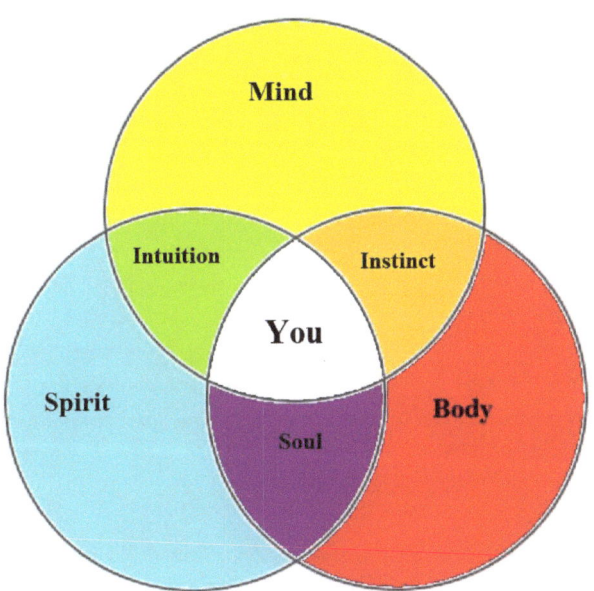

I have included this diagram to demonstrate the interdependence of the Spirit, Body, and Mind. Reality is probably more complex than this, but this is a good place to begin.

It's easy to see that Spirit, Body, and Mind are all connected. A change in the health of one part will induce a change in the health of the other parts. Your authentic self lives in Spirit. Your action lives in Body. Your volition lives in Mind.

As an example, if you do something NOT in agreement with your authentic self, a cascade effect can occur. Your Mind is diminished by that amount that is also Spirit (green in the diagram) because Spirit is not in what you're deciding to do. Since the Mind is diminished, you may suffer anger, stress, depression, or other mental dis-ease. The diminishment of the Mind will likely cause symptoms in the body allowing rashes, colds, headaches, or other dis-eases to afflict you.

As another example, let's say that you reduced a negative emotion, Fear. This would take place in your Mind. This healthy Mind growth would allow a corresponding growth in Spirit (where Love lives) and you would begin to feel greater compassion for self and others.

To use this principle in the reverse direction, if you happen to come down with the flu and want to understand why you're sick, look at your attitude, stress level, and mood, and see if you can figure out if your Mind dis-ease has been causing you to make poor dietary choices. You may have been eating a lot of ice cream for that sugar high so that you'll feel happier. Unfortunately, the excessive sugar (and possibly dairy) has now impaired your immune system, which wasn't able to defend against the flu this time around.

Watchman Nee, in his book *The Spiritual Man*, explains how the Soul is formed from the intersection of the Spirit and the Body. The Spirit communicates through the Intuition to the Mind in a way that corresponds to Mind/Body communication through the Instinct. Your self-awareness is at the center of it all.

Notably absent from this diagram is the Ego. The Ego lives in the Mind, but frequently masquerades as Intuition, Soul, Spirit, or even Instinct. In fact, it is none of these and must be brought into the center if it is to be balanced with the rest in a healthy way. For a discussion of Ego, see Eckhart Tolle, *The Power of Now*.

www.ingramcontent.com/pod-product-compliance
Lightning Source LLC
Chambersburg PA
CBHW050846290526
45792CB00002B/547